This book is dedicated to my wife, Susy, and my two sons, James and Chris, whose smiles and laughter are the very center of my happiness.

Acknowledgments

I would like to thank Dave Valent at Procter and Gamble and Ms. Sam Ton at Dr. Fresh for the information and photos they provided. Thanks also to my friend Roscel Garcia, whose advice was very helpful in the beginning stages of this text, and to my friend Dr. Michael Marfori whose insight as a children's dental specialist was very helpful in the chapter for children and brushing.

Table of Contents

Introduction

"Helping others"-two very powerful words when put together. Imagine a world based on these two words- "helping others"- there would never be war, no violence, no hunger or starvation- - people would just help one another.

I try to live my life following these two words. It's why I've written this book. Why does that child have so many cavities? Why did that teenager need so many root canals? Why did that **ADULT** need so many root canals? Why are these adults still getting lots of cavities around old fillings? How can I **HELP** other people avoid the same problems?

A lot of patients who come into my office don't realize how they are damaging their teeth. They typically admit to brushing their teeth "twice a day"- in the morning when they get up and at night before they go to bed. Guess what? In today's society, it is no longer enough- unless you are one of those people that drinks water all throughout the day and snacks to a minimum. Well, those are the patients who present with no cavities, and their teeth really are "perfect". That is less than 1% of my patient population.

Through this book I want to help people avoid getting cavities, losing teeth, developing gum disease, and spending a fortune at the dental office. *Let's face it -dentistry isn't cheap!* The high schools of this country recently changed the vending machines from soda to "sports drinks" to help control obesity. A recent study showed that sports drinks create a higher corrosive factor (acidity level) than soda. Now, instead of obese students, we'll have students walking around with cavities and needing root canals. *At least you can exercise for FREE!!!*

This book is designed as a guide to help you **PROTECT YOUR TEETH**. This book is not intended as a technical tooth repair manual. You don't need a chemistry degree to read this- there are no confusing details on molecules or complex charts. You don't have to be a rocket scientist to understand the advice. There's nothing sophisticated about the advice and there's nothing **EXPENSIVE** you need to buy. It's really a lot of common sense, adjusting some daily habits, and understanding what causes tooth decay and gum disease. There is one chapter that shows dental x-

rays with some dental anatomy but I try to simplify it as much as possible to give a basic understanding of tooth decay and bone loss(or periodontal disease).

It is also not meant as a problem solver if you have cavities. Nowadays there are several ways to fix teeth. Your local dentist can advise you as to the best way to deal with tooth decay.

Finally, it is not meant as a nutrition guide. If you need more information on eating healthy visit your local book store. There's usually a "health and nutrition" section where you can find a good book.

Thank you for taking time to read this guide- your teeth will benefit greatly if you put this advice to good use. Don't forget- ***PROTECT THOSE TEETH!!!***

Eso Tiu, DMD

"Ignore your teeth and they'll go away"

Chapter 1
The Effects of Sugared Drinks

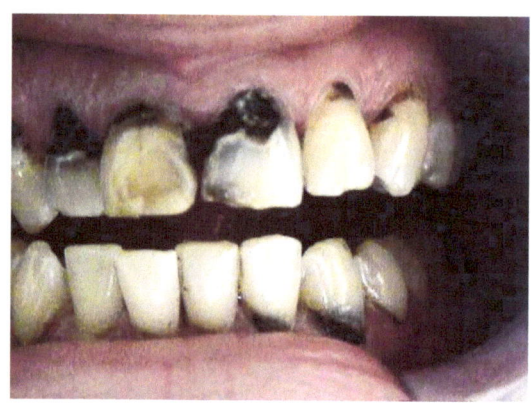

I don't meet too many people who "enjoy" going to the dentist. Most people I know actually hate going to the dentist. Usually it's due to fear, or they say: "there's no pain, so why should I go?". However, are they protecting their teeth while they don't go? Do they know what can erode the teeth, or is there gum disease setting in? There's usually no pain during the initial stages of tooth decay and gum disease. For those of you who fall into this dental phobic category, use this book as a "coaching guide" to caring for your teeth. Quite frankly, there's probably a lot of foods and drinks that you're taking that are harmful to your teeth -**but you don't know they are.** Hopefully, the pictures alone in this book will motivate you to change your daily habits. So even if you continue to not go to the dentist, you will give your teeth the best fighting chance for **SURVIVAL OVER TIME.**

Look at the photo on page 6. What was this guy's problem? "You'll never see me in the office without a cup of coffee in one of my hands- light and sweet". Imagine that- ALL DAY LONG this guy was BATHING his teeth in sugar and cream. Sure, he drinks most of it, but a lot of it is lingering around the mouth wreaking havoc and destruction through acid formation. This individual literally eroded his teeth away. How could this be prevented? Brush after EVERY CUP OF COFFEE if it has SUGAR!! That may sound unrealistic- but what are the choices here? Brush teeth to protect them or let sugar erode them away? Hmmm...

Look at the close up photo. This is just pure erosion acting constantly throughout the day over many years. This individual said he brushed twice a day- in the morning and at night. Do you think it was enough? He needs to brush after every cup of coffee because of the sugar content.

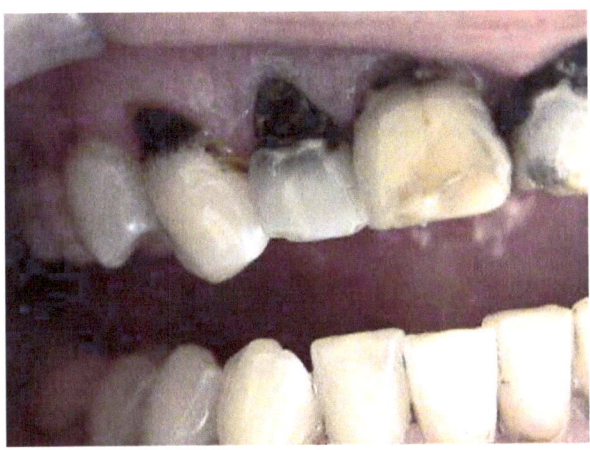

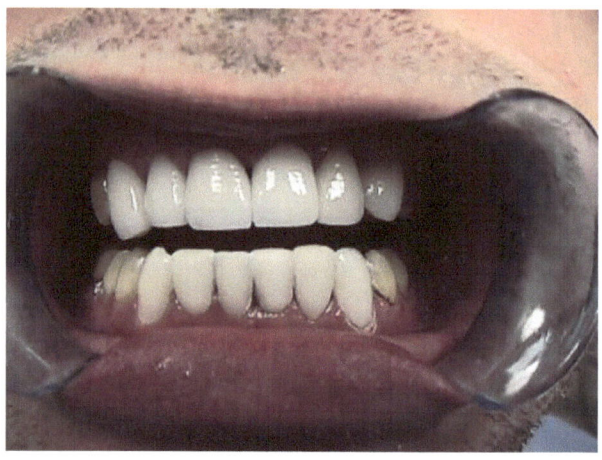

Sure, several thousand dollars later the dentist was able to make his teeth look normal again. How much does it cost to brush your teeth after any sugared beverage? **THINK ABOUT IT!!!**

If you really want to protect and preserve your teeth, don't give sugar the chance to erode them.

That leads me to **Dr. Tiu's #1 rule:** Brush after any sugared drink- soda, iced tea, sports drinks, coffee/tea with sugar...you get the idea! I don't care if you have to brush 10 times a day! PROTECT THOSE TEETH!

Bring a toothbrush to work if you have to. If you're always on the go, carry mouthwash with you and rinse out after having these drinks. Some of the big companies, like CREST, put out toothpastes and fluoride rinses to help protect against "acid wear".

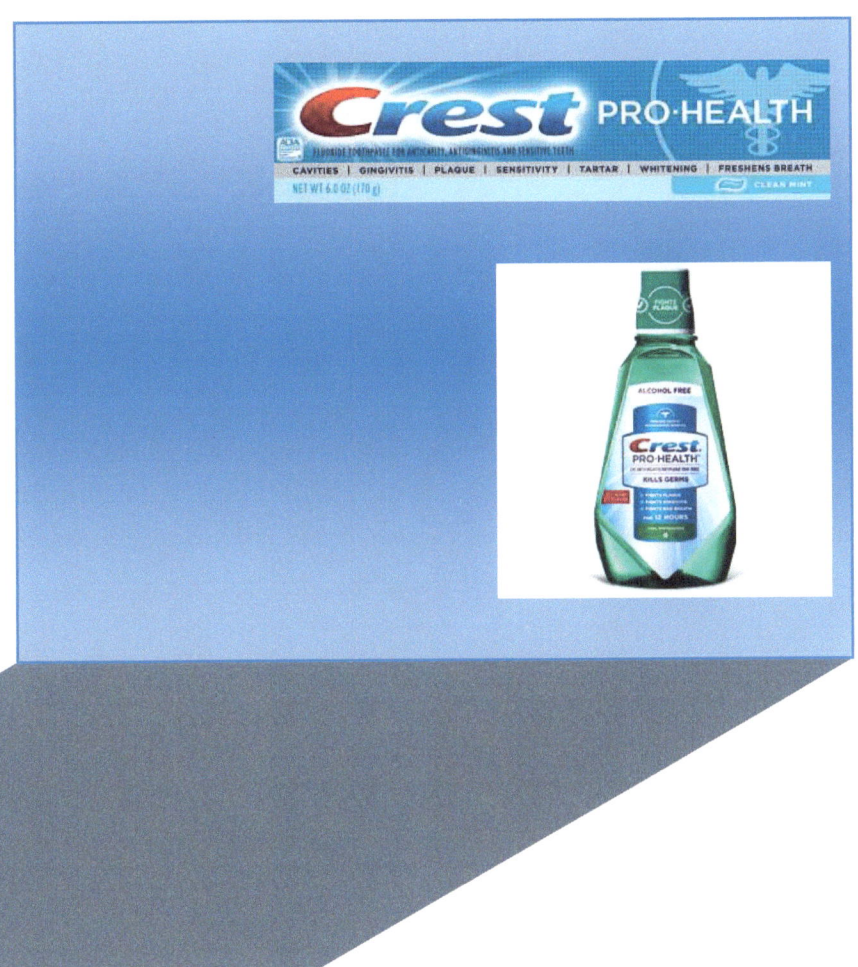

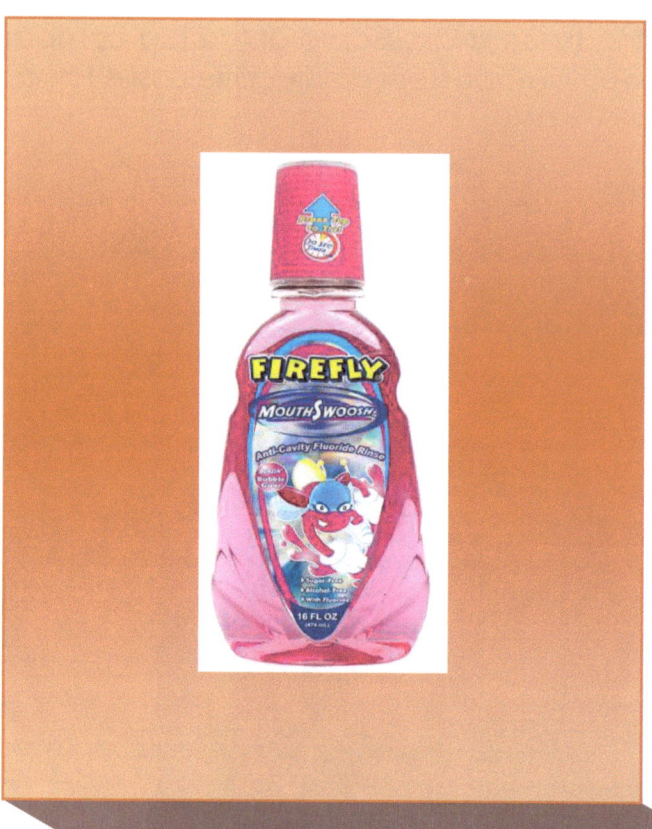

    Did you ever hear the saying "don't pour soda on your car". What will happen? The paint will erode due to the acid effect. The same thing happens to your teeth. Leave soda (or other sugar filled beverages) on your teeth and you will slowly erode your teeth over time.

    Even diet soda will cause acid formation. It just does it slower than regular soda. So don't think you're safe just because you drink diet soda. Always brush afterwards.

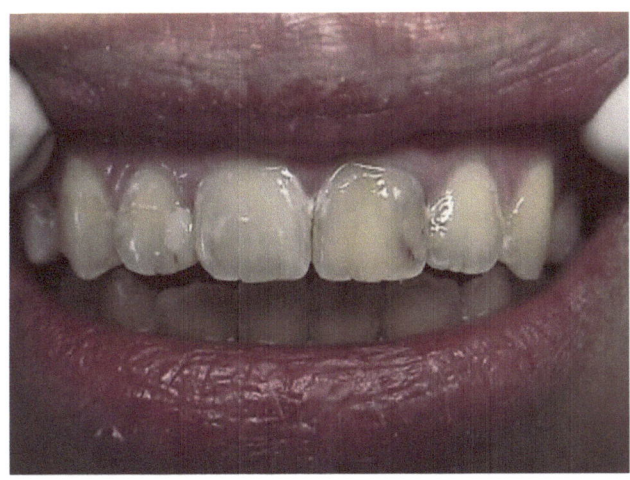

What happened here? This is a seventeen year-old who needed 4 root canals. Let's reemphasize that- **4 ROOT CANALS AT THE AGE OF SEVENTEEN!!** That did not include several other deep fillings that are potential root canals in the future! Of course I asked her -"Why all the decay?". Her first response was "I don't know". When asked about her diet she said "I eat skittles and have Coca cola for breakfast". Her mother was out of the house by 5:00a.m. as part of her work schedule. This teen formulated her own breakfast!! Going to the dentist was also not a priority EVER in her life. She only appeared in my office one day because of a toothache.

This leads me **to Dr. Tiu's #2 rule:** visit your dentist regularly for checkups and cleanings.

If your dentist says you have cavities make sure you take care of them. Waiting for something to hurt usually indicates something more involved (and much more expensive) than a regular "filling" that can solve the initial problem.

This individual obviously needed diet counseling. Interestingly, she was not aware that the candy/soda combo would destroy her teeth.

Chapter 2
Should I Stop Eating Candy?

Did you see the movie "Charlie and the Chocolate Factory"? They sure did a good job of making the dentist/orthodontist public enemy no.1 for all Halloween loving kids (and what child doesn't love Halloween?).

I think it's unrealistic to expect kids (or anyone) to stop eating candy just because the "dentist told you".

This leads me **to Dr. Tiu's #3 rule:** brush after any candy or snack- this INCLUDES "FRUIT SNACKS" which are very sticky. Like rule #1, keep sugar off the teeth.

My advice is to just brush right after you have any candy. ***This includes "fruit snacks". If you can't brush right away (or within 30 minutes), that's when you shouldn't have it.***

I love candy myself and I drink regular soda (I hate diet soda!). But, I brush after every candy bar or can of soda. You've got to keep the sugar off the teeth. I still get my sugar fix, but I also make sure I protect the teeth.

No one is immune to the effects of acid wear from sugar- it is what it is- there's no changing what it does. However, you can protect your teeth by physically removing it with a toothbrush and toothpaste.

This is an example of just changing part of your daily habits.

I had a patient who literally told me she "started having chocolate bars for breakfast". Well, as expected, she also had **5 NEW cavities, 3 of which were very deep.** "Do you brush after the chocolate?" I asked. "I brush in the morning when I wake up, and at night before I go to sleep". Sure, it's twice a day like a toothpaste label might indicate, but it's at the **WRONG TIME!!** Think about it- what good is that morning brush when shortly after you're just going to coat your teeth with chocolate? The toothpaste doesn't magically remove the sugar from the chocolate; it **doesn't BULLETPROOF your teeth.** Many people seem to feel this way. If you're going to only brush twice a day no matter what anyone says, then try brushing **after** breakfast and right after dinner.

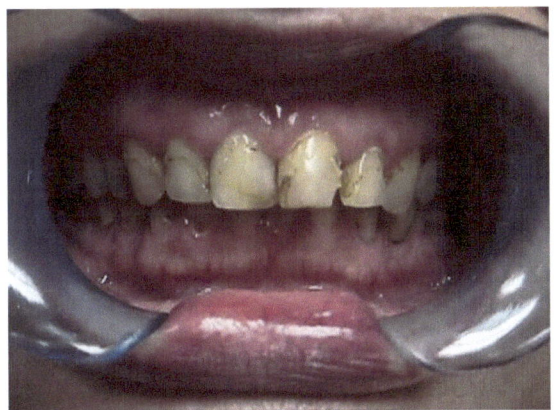

Acid erosion all over the front teeth

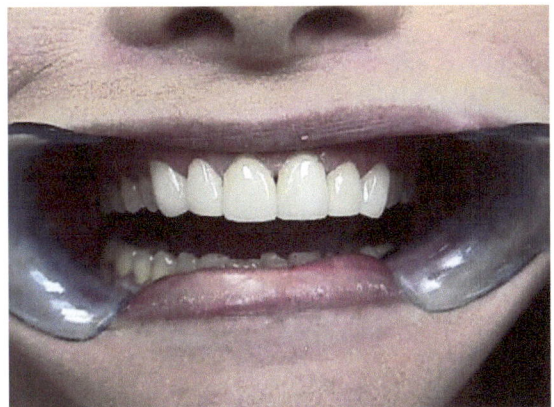

Expensive repair to look normal again.

"We're all employees of our children"

Chapter 3
Children and Brushing

This is where it all starts. Like with anything else, good brushing habits should be taught from childhood.

I truly believe there can be a "cavity free" school someday if parents just take the time to brush their children's teeth after snacks or have them brush their own teeth after all snacks when they're old enough. It doesn't take that much time, and it's a good investment over time. How much does it cost to fix your child's teeth when they need fillings or root canals, or whatever? Even with insurance, it can still cost a pretty penny.

How hard do you want to work just to fix cavities on your child's teeth? Let's rephrase that- ***how much of your extra spending money do you want to give up fixing your children's teeth?***

What if they didn't need those fillings or root canals? What could you do with the extra money? How much does it cost to brush your child's teeth after any snack? ***Think about it!*** True, a lot of parents are not home with their children during the day to keep after their brushing habits. Well, then whoever is home with them (grandma, the nanny, the babysitter, etc.) should have specific instructions to make sure they brush those teeth after all snacks. Hopefully, by the time the kids are old enough to be on their own, *they'll want to keep their own teeth clean.* How about a mandatory "brushing period " for schools since all the soda machines were changed to "sports drink" machines? (Again, these drinks have been shown to have a higher corrosive factor than soda).

Make brushing fun for them. There are so many brushes with characters and blinking lights, spinning brushes, and brushes that make noise. Let them "choose their weapon". They will enjoy it more that way.

I'm always guiding my two sons to brush after snacks, juices, candy, etc...So far, at 5 and 7 years old they have no cavities. If your child has no cavities right now, that's great-keep going. *Keep those teeth protected! They can grow up cavity free with your guidance, and you WILL save a lot of money!!(As well as the beautiful smile on your child's face.)*

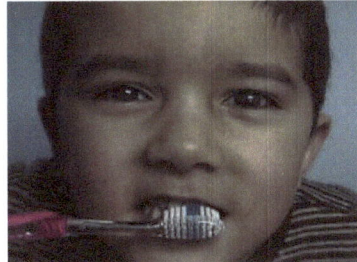 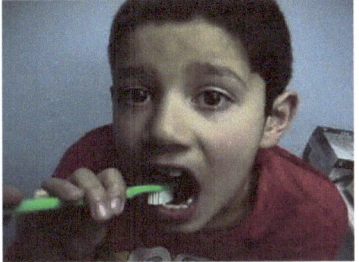

Brush those front teeth! Here's a hint: make sure to TIP the brush up so it can reach BEHIND those lower front teeth (see photo on right). This is a commonly missed area.

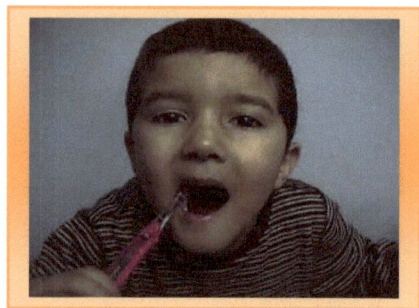
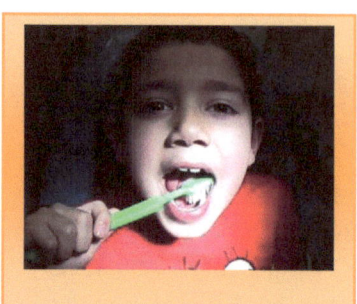

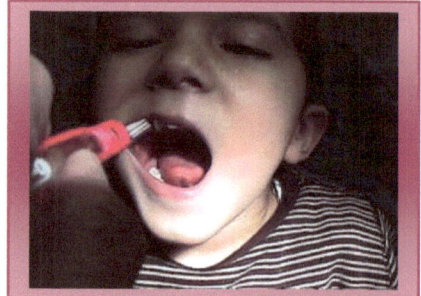
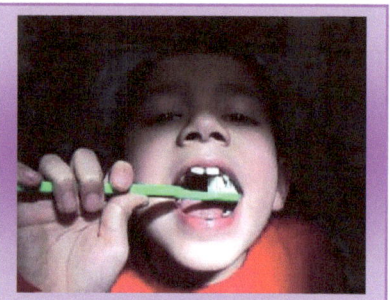

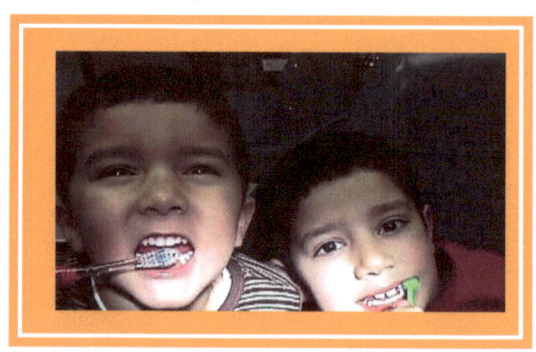

Brushing your child's teeth is not difficult. It's like cleaning your car. Scrub all surfaces. If they've eaten cookies or some other snack with a lot of debris, try having them rinse out first several times to get rid of the excess particles. If they've eaten something very sticky like raisins, peanut brittle, fruit snacks, etc., then you might have to brush several times. These are the most dangerous snacks because they physically stick to the teeth and can cause rapid acid erosion (cavity formation) on the enamel(outer hard surface of teeth). Try to keep these to a minimum or eliminate these kind altogether.

Fluoride

Have your children use a daily fluoride rinse. It will help make the teeth more resistant to cavity formation. The following is one popular example.

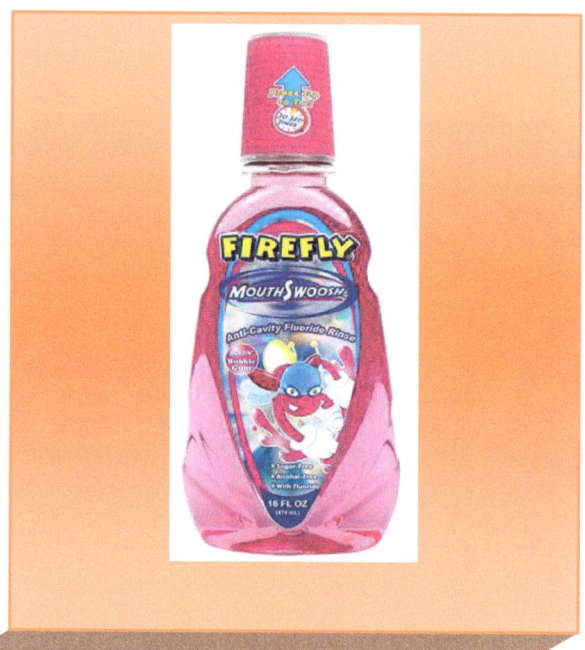

Dr. Fresh makes the **"Firefly" brand.** These are excellent products for children. They have their own line of toothbrushes, toothpaste, and fluoride. Each product comes with its own built-in light timer that blinks for a specified amount of time depending on which product is being used. Again, this is something that makes oral hygiene **FUN** for kids. See the appendix for additional information .

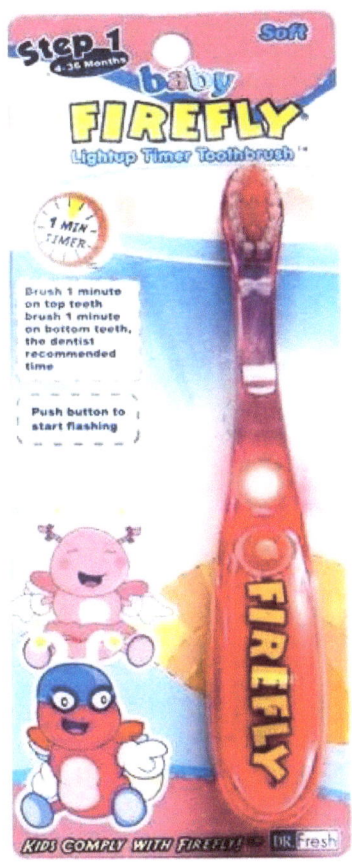

Brushing for baby

"First visit by first birthday" is a recommendation by the American Academy of Pediatric Dentistry. You want to start a prevention routine right from the start. Expectant mothers are advised to visit their pediatricians before the birth of their child. I think it's a good idea to also include a pediatric dental specialist. Dental problems like "baby bottle decay"(Early Childhood Caries) can be avoided by visiting your dental specialist ahead of time. Once your baby has teeth only water should be in a bottle while sleeping. Letting them fall asleep with juice or milk in a bottle will invariably lead to rampant decay all over-"baby bottle decay". It may take a few nights of crying during the adjustment but this will be well worth the effort-your child will maintain a beautiful cavity free smile! Visit the website for the American Academy of Pediatric Dentists and click on Parent Resource Center for more excellent advice.

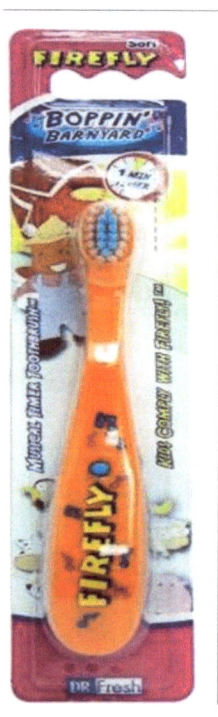

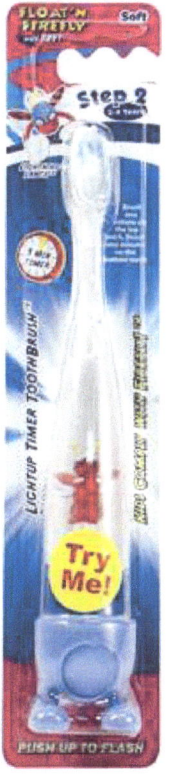
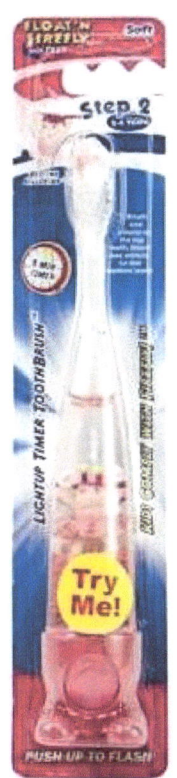
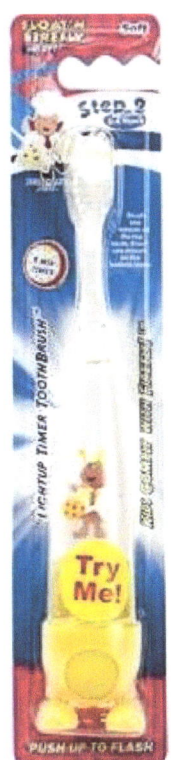

Variety makes brushing fun!

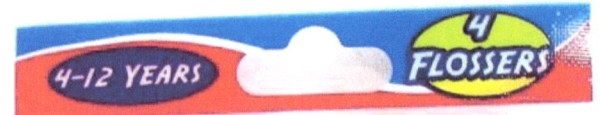

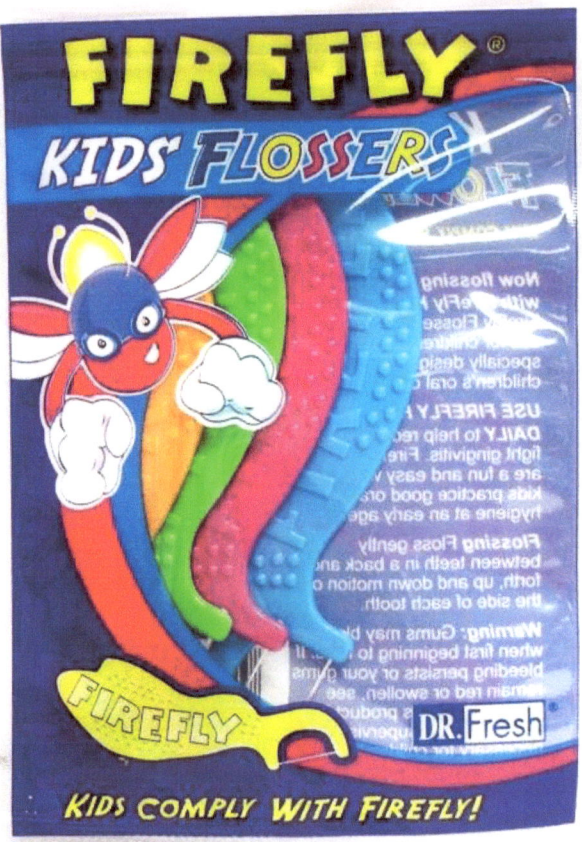

Here's a great way to start your kids flossing!

Chapter 4
Mouthguards- Why They're Important

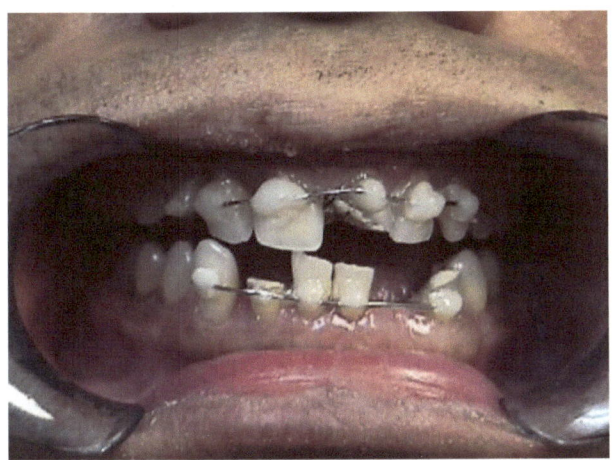

This photo speaks for itself. This patient was a victim of a raquetball accident. The side of his opponent's racket hit him square in the mouth, knocking out a few teeth on the bottom and fracturing several others. Needless to say this person needed several root canals, crowns and several thousand dollars to repair **what could've been prevented, or minimized with an inexpensive mouth guard.**

Don't play around!! If you're involved in sports with potential hard physical contact invest in a mouth guard! You can buy one in the store, or for a little more, you can have a custom fit mouth guard made by your local dentist. Either way it's worth the investment.

Chapter 5
Understanding Dental X-rays: basic concepts

The purpose of this chapter is to familiarize you with dental x-rays. What is the dentist looking at? What do the teeth look like? What are those white spots on the teeth? Again, this is just a simple overview. Your dentist will review your x-rays with you at your regular check-up. After reading this section, you will be able to understand better what he or she is trying to show you.

When you view dental x-rays, imagine the person is facing you. Let's look at our model, "Harry the skull", in the following page. The photos show three different views: right side of face, straight on view, and left side of face.

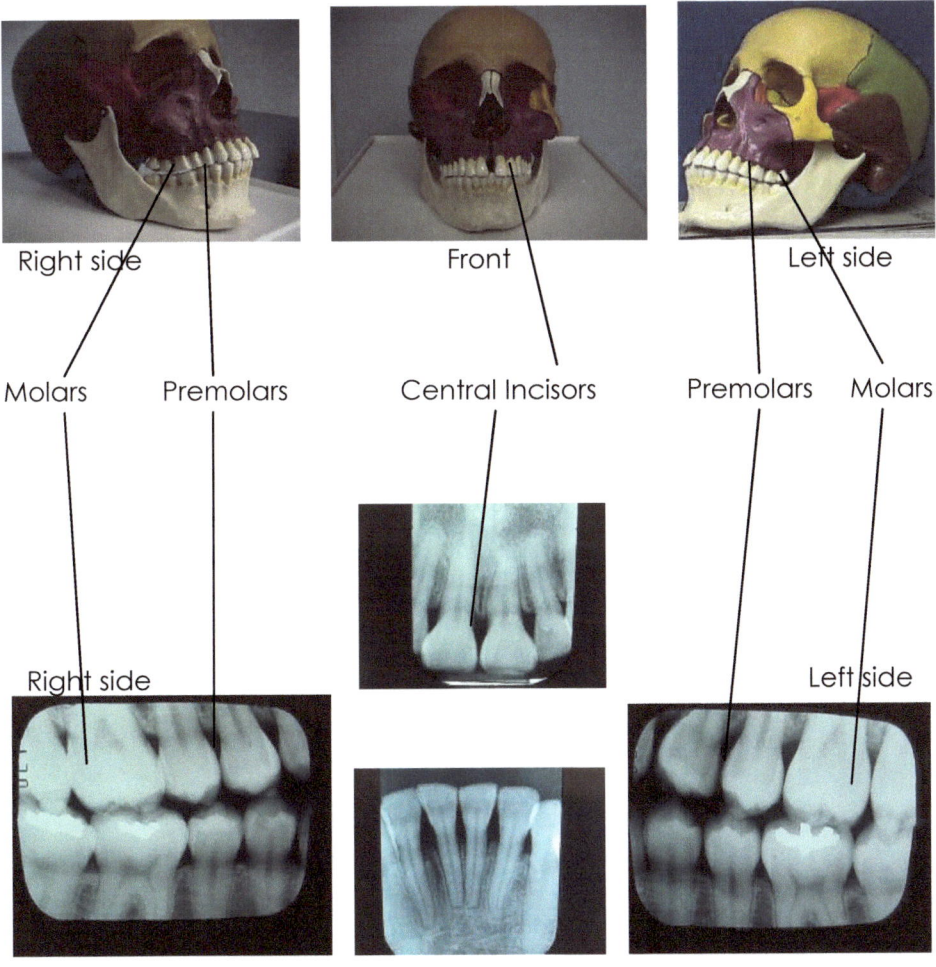

Right side

Front

Left side

Molars

Premolars

Central Incisors

Premolars

Molars

Right side

Left side

So what's in a dental x-ray? You can see different layers of a tooth, the nerve inside , and the bone surrounding it. You can also see fillings and cavities. Just remember this: the harder (or denser) something is, the lighter it will show on an x-ray. Let's look at some examples.

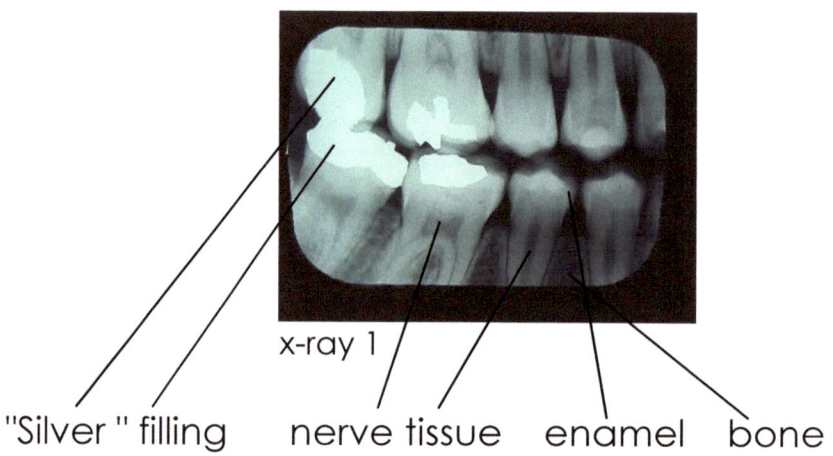

x-ray 1

"Silver " filling   nerve tissue   enamel   bone

Note the "silver" filling- it's a type of metal. It's so dense and solid so it shows up as a "white" area on the x-ray. By contrast, look at the nerve tissue. This is a soft, less dense material so it shows up as a "darker" area inside the tooth. There is the outer tooth layer-the enamel, and there's the bone surrounding the tooth.

Let's see another example

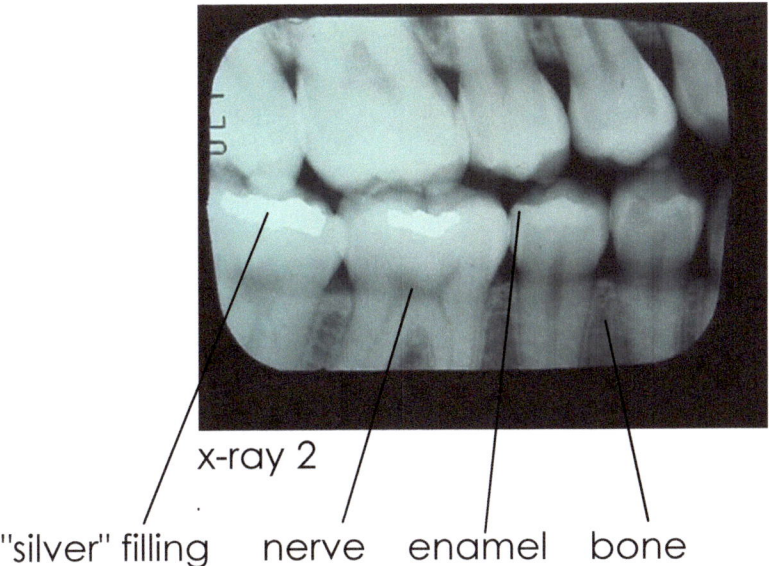

x-ray 2

"silver" filling   nerve   enamel   bone

Just for fun, let's check out an x-ray with the entire tooth in the image.

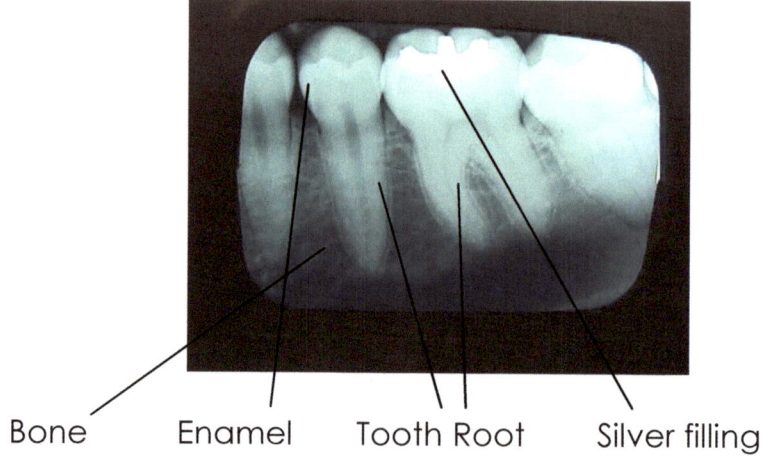

Bone   Enamel   Tooth Root   Silver filling

Next we'll look at x-rays with dental problems. The following x-rays are from an **18-year old patient** who had a "sweet tooth". When asked about her intake of soda, iced tea, or candy, she smiled and said "all the above". When asked about brushing she said, "I brush when I get up in the morning, and before I go to bed". Let's look at the extensive damage to her teeth.

Cavities(holes) forming in between the teeth

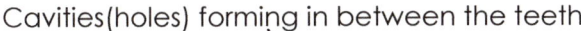

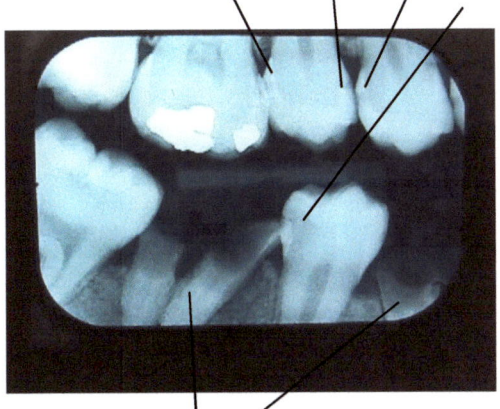

What happened to these teeth? Where are they? They've eroded away thanks to heavy sugar intake and not brushing right after. These are just roots left in the bone.

Again, the same patient. Look at the severe erosion and destruction this teen is doing to herself –**without realizing!!**

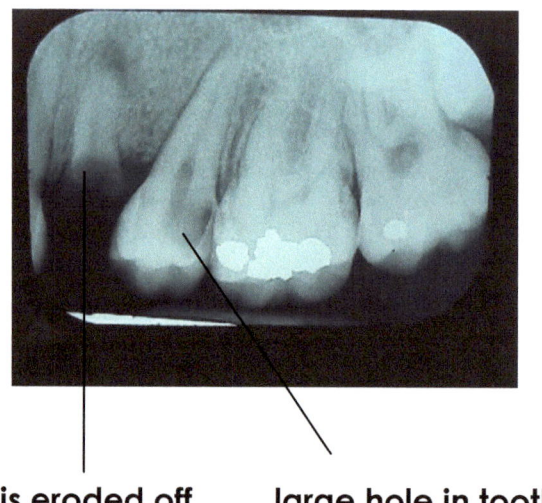

Tooth is eroded off   **large hole in tooth**

Chapter 6: Gum Disease

Gum disease, or periodontitis, is the loss of bone around teeth. As a result the teeth become loose, and ultimately need to be removed, or extracted. It generally progresses over many years-it is a "slow" disease process. That's actually the only good thing about it. The bad thing about it is YOU MAY HAVE IT BUT AREN'T AWARE. That's because in the early stages there are no symptoms (there's usually no pain). If you never visit the dentist, you may not know you have gum disease until it's in the advanced stages. This is when you may suddenly realize your teeth are loose, or your gums have pain and swelling, or your gums bleed spontaneously or while brushing, or everyone covers their face when they talk to you because your breath smells horrific. If you let your teeth get to this stage it may be too late to save them.

So what causes this "silent" tooth killer? Simply put, gum disease is caused by food particles and bacteria accumulating and hardening(or calcifying)around the teeth at the gum level(on the roots). The body's natural response to this hardened layer of bacteria and food attached to the teeth is to "run away" from it- the bone "runs away" from the tooth. As it slowly disappears, food particles and bacteria "chase" it. As more tooth is exposed, the bacteria and food particles simply settle deeper into the "pockets" created from the bone disappearing. And the cycle continues over time: bone runs away, bacteria follow, bone runs away, bacteria follow, etc...So how do you stop the process? You generally have two options-you can remove the calcified bacteria/food layer on the roots, or you can remove the tooth altogether. Let's look at these options.

1. **Remove the calcified bacteria/food layer**: If you want your teeth to survive, this is the way to go. Only your dental professional can do this treatment. This is generally not treated with just a regular "cleaning". You need to have what's known as a "deep cleaning". This type of cleaning is a little more involved. The bacteria layer has to be scraped off the root surface of the tooth with special instruments. Anesthetic is also generally required so you don't feel anything (otherwise it can be quite painful). These special cleanings are also performed in sections-usually one side at a time. As I said above, gum disease is a slow process. This is another reason to follow Dr. Tiu's rule #2- make regular visits to the dentist. (Actually, if you have been going regularly, then you should never have gum disease-EVER!). If it is caught early, you might only have to go through the deep cleaning once, and then just maintain your regular cleanings and checkups with your dentist to make sure it doesn't recur. If it is caught in the later stages you may need multiple phases of treatment.

   Once the bone disappears, **it does not come back**-even if the disease process is removed!

This leads me to **Dr. Tiu's rule #4:** If your dental professional recommends a "deep cleaning" because you're showing signs of early gum disease, do this ASAP-everyday you delay means that much more disease and bone loss .

2. **Removing or extracting the tooth/teeth**: This seems like a simple solution- remove tooth or teeth with bacteria and don't worry about it anymore. There are a lot of people with this mentality. Some people say, "I'll just wear dentures like my grandmother (or mother)". So let's think that through just a little more. How do denture wearers maintain their dentures? They have to remove them at night and soak them in water to let the gums rest and clean or condition the denture. Think about that-when you wake up every day, do you want to see your teeth soaking in a cup of water? Are you going to feel good about that? Worse yet, a lot of denture wearers can't eat OR taste their food normally. A denture is a huge piece of plastic with artificial teeth that covers most of your hard dental tissue-it's not part of your body- *IT'S ARTIFICIAL!* It also moves around when you try to eat. Do you really want to go that way??!!!! **THINK ABOUT IT!!**

Look at the following x-rays(if necessary, review chapter 5 to familiarize yourself with the basic features of the dental x-ray).

Let's compare a case of someone with very good bone versus someone with bone loss, or **PERIODONTITIS**:

The x-rays on the left are a patient with good bone. Note how the bone surrounds all the teeth. If this patient brushes regularly, and maintain the teeth properly, he should keep all his teeth **the rest of his life.**

Now look at the x-rays on the right. This is a case of severe gum disease. What are those white bumps coming off the side of the tooth roots? That's calcified bacteria and food particles- *it's so thick it shows up on the dental x-ray!* Look at the bone level. The body doesn't like this layer of bacteria so it is "running away". This is the result of years of accumulation Some of these teeth can't be saved. Look at the "floater" tooth-there's almost no bone support around it.

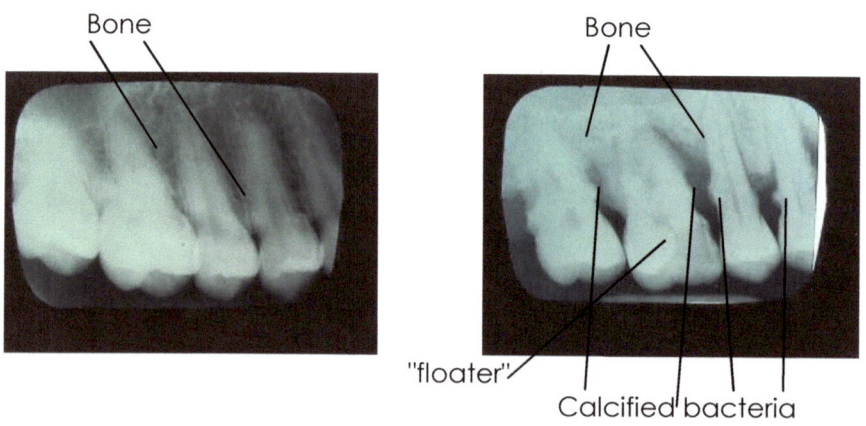

Bone   Bone

"floater"

Calcified bacteria

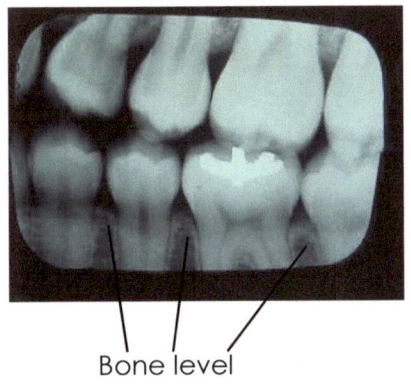

Bone level

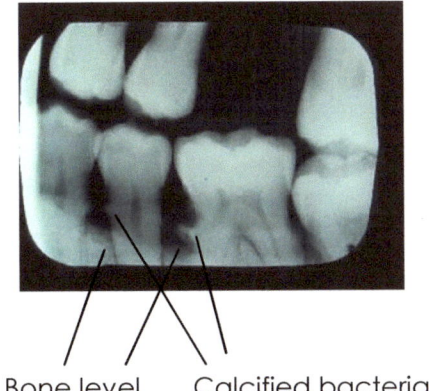

Bone level   Calcified bacteria

Just a few final notes:

a) Notice that most of the teeth have **NO CAVITIES.** So you can have cavity free teeth growing up and STILL LOSE YOUR TEETH to gum disease. This is another reason to follow Dr. Tiu's rule #2!!

b) This is where **FLOSSING** is very important. A toothbrush cannot reach in between teeth. When you floss, make sure you move the floss **UP AND DOWN. Don't "shoe shine" it** (back and forth). A lot of people make this mistake.

Chapter 7: Smile!

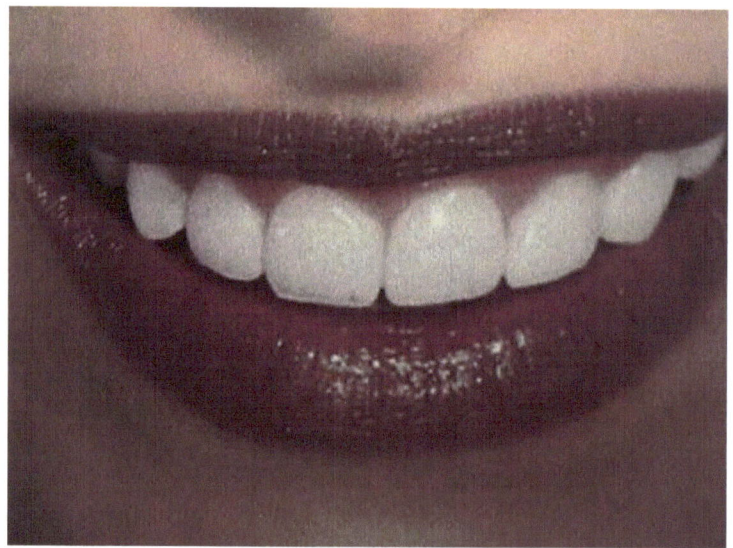

"A smile takes but a moment, but the memory of it lasts forever."

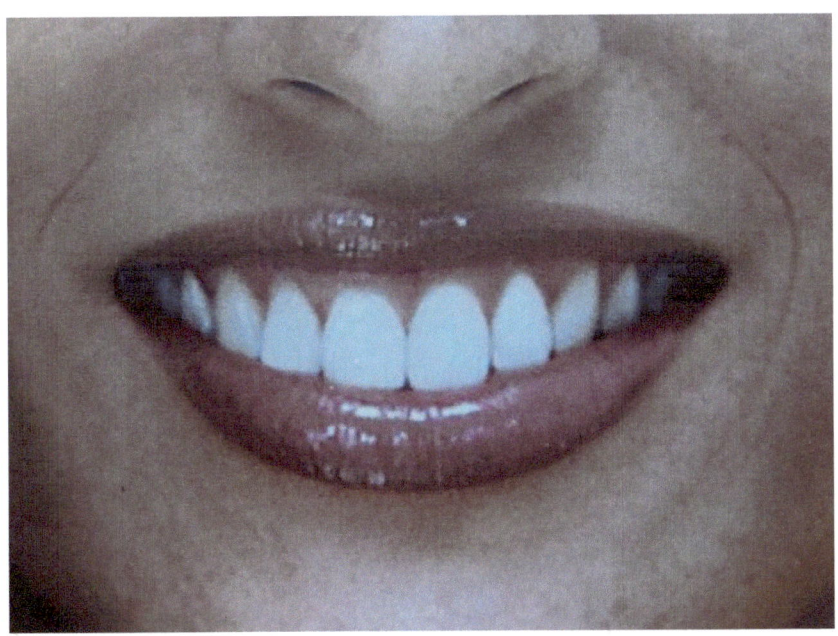

"Keep a smile on your face and let your personality be your autograph."

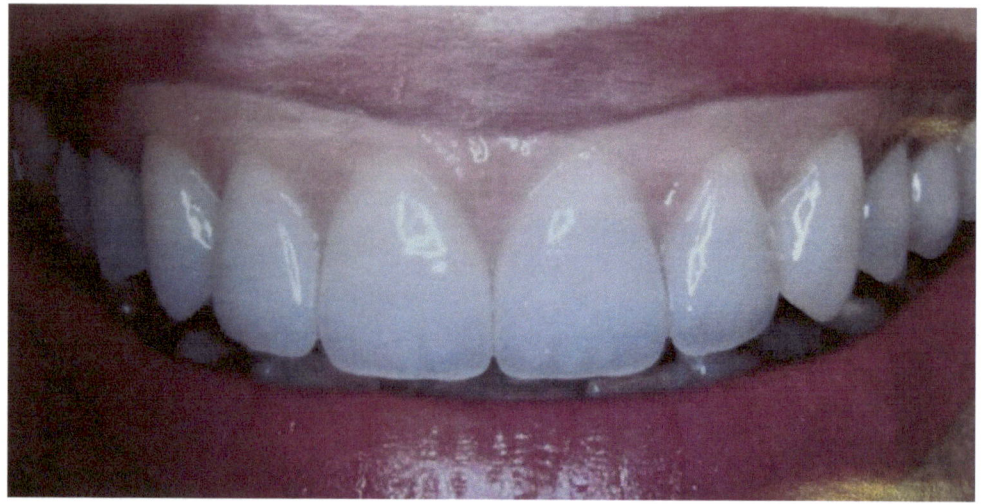

"If you haven't seen your wife smile at a traffic cop, you haven't seen her smile her prettiest." (You see! A nice smile really does come in handy once in awhile...)

Appendix 1

FLUORIDE RINSE BY DR. FRESH®
Fact Sheet

What's better than an anti-cavity fluoride rinse for giving kids that extra protection they need against cavities? An anti-cavity fluoride rinse that's pretty in pink, and pleasing in taste. Of course, it also has to be free of sugar and alcohol but full of fun! **FIREFLY® MOUTHSWOOSH™ ANTI-CAVITY FLUORIDE RINSE by DR. FRESH®** *delivers on all counts.*

- Contains fluoride to help prevent cavities

- Attracts kids with its bright pink color and light-up timer cap

- LCD light in cap incorporates "blinking technology" to flash brightly for thirty seconds when filled with liquid

- 30-second flashing time promotes proper and effective rinsing; rinse is spit out when the light goes out. 30 seconds is the dentist-recommended rinse time.

- Developed for ages 6 and up

- Alcohol-free

- Sugar-free

- Bubble-gum flavored with great kid appeal

- Used once daily after brushing under parental supervision

- Refrain from eating and drinking for 30 minutes after use

- SRP $4.99, www.drfresh.com

- Available at mass merchandise stores like Target, Wal-Mart, Walgreens, Rite Aid and www.drugstore.com

- For more information, contact Megan Brown at Light Years Ahead at (323)650-2201 or at megn@lightyearsahead.com

Appendix 2

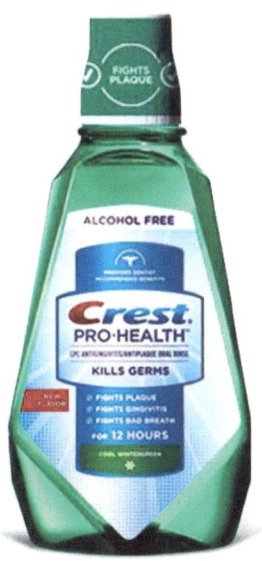

For those who are interested, to aid in optimizing oral health, Crest has developed the "paste-brush-rinse night regimen". You can obtain more information by visiting http://www.dentalcare.com. Click the "Product Research" sub-heading and search under "Regimen" for the topic and "Gerlach" as the author.

Brushing Tips

1. Use a SOFT bristle brush. Avoid HARD brushes- these can wear away your enamel rapidly.
2. Don't brush hard. Brush gently, but brush thoroughly.
3. Brush all surfaces-outside, inside, and on top-of all teeth. For the lower front teeth, angle the brush handle up to reach behind.
4. For optimal oral health, brush right after eating.

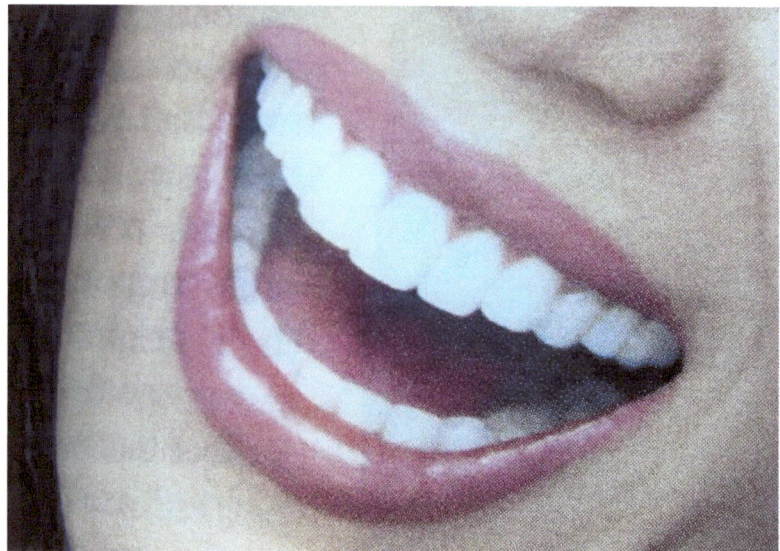

Closing Thoughts

Location, location, location…soda spill on the table, who cares; left over iced tea in a cup, so what; sports drink getting poured on coach's head, nice going; BUT- soda, iced tea, or sports drink on the teeth? That's BAD!! Get it outta' there! Brush it off! Wake up America! Be more conscious of what's sitting on your teeth. If you're taking in sweets all day then you better be brushing all day. Just because you need to drink something all day to stay awake, don't take it out on your teeth.

I hope in reading this book and in following the recommendations the occurrence of cavities and gum disease in all individuals will decrease significantly. But everyone must do their part. Parents, start teaching your children; teachers and coaches, start teaching your students to brush or rinse out after sports drinks. If you haven't been to the dentist consider having a checkup- if not for cavities, then to check the condition of your gums and keep gum disease away forever.

You can do it-I know you can. Remember- **PROTECT THOSE TEETH!!**

About the Author

Eso Tiu, DMD graduated from the University of Medicine and Dentistry of New Jersey in 1994. He maintains a private practice in Bergen County, NJ. If you have any questions or comments you can send an e-mail to Esofine@aol.com.

Notes

Notes